Ivosic

 of Immunology based on the material in this book
Further information may be obtained from:
sby Company
ine Industrial Drive, St. Louis, MO63146

IMMUNOLO

A Slide Atla
is available.
The C.V. Mc
11830 West

IMMUNOLOGY

IVAN M. ROITT
MA DSc(Oxon) FRCPath FRS

Professor and Head of Department
of Immunology
The Middlesex Hospital Medical School
London W1

JONATHAN BROSTOFF
MA DM(Oxon) FRCP FRCPath

Reader in Clinical Immunology
Department of Immunology
The Middlesex Hospital Medical School
London W1

DAVID K. MALE
MA PhD

Research Associate
Department of Immunology
The Middlesex Hospital Medical School
London W1

The C. V. Mosby Company · St Louis · Toronto

Gower Medical Publishing · London · New York · 1985

DISTRIBUTORS

USA and Mexico
The C. V. Mosby Company
11830 Westline Industrial Drive, St. Louis, MO63146

Canada
The C. V. Mosby Company Ltd
120 Melford Drive, Toronto, Ontario M1B 2X5

Japan
Nankodo Company Limited.
42-6, Hongo 3-chome, Bunkyo, Tokyo 113

All other Countries
Churchill Livingstone
Medical Division of Longman Group Limited,
Robert Stevenson House, 1-3 Baxter's Place,
Leith Walk, Edinburgh EH1 3AF

British Library Cataloguing in Publication Data
Roitt, Ivan M.
 Immunology
 I. Immunology
 I. Title   II. Brostoff, Jonathan
 III. Male, David K.
 574.2'9   QR181

ISBN 0 – 906923 – 35 – 2 (Gower)
    0 – 443 – 029121 (Churchill Livingstone)

Library of Congress Cataloging in Publication Data
Roitt, Ivan Maurice
 Immunology
 Bibliography: p.
 Includes index.
 1. Immunology. I Brostoff, Jonathan.
 II. Male, David K., 1954-   . III. Title.
 QR181.R58 1985 616.07'9 85-750

ISBN 0 – 906923 – 35 – 2

Printed in Hong Kong by Mandarin Offset International

Contents

Preface   viii
Acknowledgements   viii

1 Adaptive and Innate Immunity

THE INNATE IMMUNE SYSTEM   1.1
  Phagocytes 1.2, NK Cells and Soluble Factors 1.2
INFLAMMATION   1.3
  Chemotaxis 1.4, Phagocytosis 1.4
ANTIBODY – A FLEXIBLE ADAPTOR   1.5
ANTIGEN   1.6
ADAPTIVE IMMUNITY AND CLONAL SELECTION   1.6
INTEGRATED DEFENCE MECHANISMS   1.7
VACCINATION   1.9
IMMUNOPATHOLOGY   1.9

2 Cells Involved in the Immune Response

LYMPHOID CELLS   2.2
  Morphological Heterogeneity of Lymphocytes 2.2, T Cells 2.2,
  B Cells 2.4, Lymphocyte Proliferation and Maturation 2.5
'NULL' OR 'THIRD POPULATION' CELLS   2.8
MONONUCLEAR PHAGOCYTIC SYSTEM (MONOCYTES)   2.8
  The Reticuloendothelial System 2.8, Antigen-Presenting
  Cells 2.10
THE POLYMORPHONUCLEAR GRANULOCYTES   2.12
  (POLYMORPHS)
  Neutrophils 2.12, Eosinophils 2.13, Basophils and
  Mast Cells 2.13, Platelets 2.14
SUMMARY   2.15

3 The Lymphoid System

  Primary and Secondary Lymphoid Tissue 3.1
PRIMARY LYMPHOID ORGANS   3.1
  The Thymus 3.1, The Bursa of Fabricius and its
  Mammalian Equivalent 3.2
SECONDARY LYMPHOID ORGANS   3.2
  The Spleen 3.3, Lymph Nodes and the Lymphatic system 3.4,
  Mucosal Associated Lymphoid Tissue (MALT) 3.7
LYMPHOCYTE RECIRCULATION   3.8

4 Major Histocompatibility Complex

INHERITANCE OF MHC GENES   4.1
  Inbred Mouse Strains 4.1
ARRANGEMENT OF MHC GENES   4.2
CELLULAR DISTRIBUTION OF MHC ANTIGENS   4.3
RECOMBINATION BETWEEN INBRED STRAINS   4.3
STRUCTURAL VARIATION IN MHC ANTIGENS – PUBLIC AND   4.3
  PRIVATE SPECIFICITIES
  Tissue Typing 4.4
CURRENTLY RECOGNIZED HLA SPECIFICITIES AND   4.5
  LINKAGE DISEQUILIBRIUM
STRUCTURE OF THE MHC ANTIGENS   4.6
FUNCTIONS OF THE MHC ANTIGENS   4.8

5 Antibody Structure and Function

THE FIVE IMMUNOGLOBULIN CLASSES   5.1
ANTIBODY FUNCTION   5.1
IMMUNOGLOBULIN CLASSES AND SUBCLASSES   5.2
THE OCCURRENCE AND PHYSICOCHEMICAL PROPERTIES   5.2
  OF IMMUNOGLOBULINS

ANTIBODY STRUCTURE   5.3
THE GENETIC BASIS OF ANTIBODY HETEROGENEITY   5.6
  Isotypic Variation 5.6, Allotypic Variation 5.6,
  Idiotypic Variation 5.6
ANTIBODY EFFECTOR FUNCTIONS   5.6
STRUCTURE IN RELATION TO FUNCTION   5.7
STRUCTURE IN RELATION TO ANTIGEN BINDING   5.8

6 Antigen-Antibody Reactions

ANTIGEN-ANTIBODY BINDING   6.1
ANTIBODY AFFINITY   6.2
AFFINITY AND AVIDITY   6.2
ANTIBODY SPECIFICITY   6.3
THE PHYSIOLOGICAL SIGNIFICANCE OF HIGH AND   6.5
  LOW AFFINITY ANTIBODIES
DETERMINATION OF AFFINITY AND AVIDITY   6.5
ANTIBODY AFFINITY HETEROGENEITY   6.5

7 Complement

THE COMPLEMENT PROTEINS   7.2
  Proteins of the Classical Pathway 7.2, Proteins of the
  Alternative Pathway 7.2
A PRIMITIVE COMPLEMENT SYSTEM   7.3
COMPARISON OF THE CLASSICAL AND ALTERNATIVE   7.3
  PATHWAYS
THE CLASSICAL COMPLEMENT PATHWAY   7.4
  Fixation of C1 by Immunoglobulin 7.4, Fixation and
  Activation of C4 and C2 by the C1qrs Complex 7.5,
  Action of the C4b2b Complex on C3 to form C4b2b3b 7.6,
  Action of C3b on C5 7.6
C3b (C4b) COATINGS AND IMMUNEADHERENCE   7.6
ANAPHYLATOXIN FORMATION   7.7
BIOLOGICAL EFFECTS OF C3a   7.8
BIOLOGICAL EFFECTS OF C5a   7.8
ASSEMBLY OF THE C5-9 MEMBRANE ATTACK COMPLEX   7.8
THE ALTERNATIVE PATHWAY   7.9
BREAKDOWN OF C3b   7.10
COBRA VENOM FACTOR (CVF) AND C3 NEPHRITIC   7.10
  FACTOR (C3 Nef)
EFFECT OF C3-9 DEPLETION ON THE ADAPTIVE IMMUNE   7.11
  RESPONSE
INHERITED COMPLEMENT DEFICIENCIES AND THEIR   7.11
  EFFECTS IN MAN
INHIBITION OF C1 AND HEREDITARY ANGIOEDEMA   7.12
COMPLEMENT AND THE MAJOR HISTOCOMPATIBILITY   7.13
  COMPLEX

8 The Antibody Response

PRIMARY AND SECONDARY ANTIBODY RESPONSES   8.1
ASSAYING ANTIBODY FORMING CELLS (AFCs) –   8.1
  THE PLAQUE ASSAY
HAPTENS AND CARRIERS   8.2
T-DEPENDENT AND T-INDEPENDENT ANTIGENS   8.3
AFFINITY MATURATION   8.4
ANTIGEN PRESENTATION   8.5
MECHANISMS OF CELL COOPERATION   8.6
T CELL FACTORS   8.7
ADJUVANTS   8.9

9 The Generation of Antibody Diversity

THEORIES OF ANTIBODY FORMATION   9.1
IMMUNOGLOBULIN VARIABILITY   9.2

LIGHT CHAIN GENE RECOMBINATION — 9.3
HEAVY CHAIN GENE RECOMBINATION — 9.5
RECOMBINATION SEQUENCES — 9.5
ADDITIONAL DIVERSITY — 9.6
    Variable Recombination 9.6, Somatic Mutation 9.6
HEAVY CHAIN CONSTANT REGION GENES — 9.8
MEMBRANE AND SECRETED IMMUNOGLOBLIN — 9.9
PRODUCTION OF IMMUNOGLOBULIN — 9.11

10 Regulation of the Immune Response

THE REGULATORY EFFECT OF ANTIBODY — 10.1
THE REGULATORY EFFECT OF IMMUNE COMPLEXES — 10.2
IDIOTYPIC REGULATION — 10.3
EVIDENCE THAT IDIOTYPIC INTERACTIONS ARE IMPORTANT IN IMMUNOREGULATION — 10.4
REGULATION BY CELLULAR MECHANISMS – SUPPRESSOR T CELLS — 10.8
CELLULAR CIRCUITS — 10.9
FUNCTION OF THE MHC IN REGULATION — 10.10
REGULATION OF THE MODE OF RESPONSE — 10.10
NON-SPECIFIC REGULATION — 10.10
SELF/NON-SELF DISCRIMINATION — 10.11

11 Cell-mediated Immunity

RECOGNITION OF ANTIGEN BY T CELLS — 11.1
MHC RESTRICTION — 11.2
T CELL RECEPTORS FOR MHC GLYCOPEPTIDES — 11.3
T CELL RECEPTORS FOR ANTIGEN — 11.3
    Gene Arrangement and Structure of the T Cell Receptor 11.4, Immunoglobulin Idiotypes 11.4
ANTIGEN-PRESENTING CELLS — 11.4
ACTIVATION OF T CELLS BY ANTIGEN-PRESENTING CELLS — 11.4
CELL-MEDIATED CYTOTOXICITY — 11.5
MHC RESTRICTED CYTOTOXIC T CELLS — 11.5
NATURAL KILLER CELLS — 11.6
    The Identity of NK Cells 11.6, Relationship of NK Cells to K Cells and Cytotoxic T Cells 11.6, Mechanism of NK Cell-Mediated Lysis 11.6
ANTIBODY-DEPENDENT CELL-MEDIATED CYTOTOXICITY (ADCC) — 11.6
THE CENTRAL ROLE OF MACROPHAGES — 11.7
    Macrophage Activation by T Lymphocyte-Derived Mediators 11.8
LYMPHOKINES — 11.8
    The Nature of Lymphokines and the Cells of Origin 11.8, The Complexity of Macrophage Activation 11.10

12 Immunological Tolerance

PATHWAYS TO TOLERANCE — 12.2
PATHWAYS TO B CELL TOLERANCE — 12.2
    Clonal Abortion 12.2, Clonal Exhaustion 12.2, Functional Deletion 12.3, Antibody Forming Cell (AFC) Blockade 12.3
PATHWAYS TO T CELL TOLERANCE — 12.3
    T-suppressors 12.3
GENERAL CHARACTERISTICS OF T CELL AND B CELL TOLERANCE — 12.3
    Induction Time 12.4, Antigen Dose 12.4, Antigen Persistence 12.4, Specificity 12.4, Duration 12.4
INCOMPLETE TOLERANCE — 12.5
    Affinity and Isotype Maturation 12.5, Humoral and Cell-Mediated Responses 12.5, Determinants 12.5, Tissue Specificity 12.5
MECHANISMS OF TOLERANCE INDUCTION — 12.6
    Antigen-Induced Tolerance 12.6, Tolerance Enhanced by Immunosuppressive Drugs 12.8, Antibody-Induced Tolerance 12.9
SELF TOLERANCE — 12.10
TOLERANCE IN AREAS OF POTENTIAL THERAPEUTIC APPLICATION — 12.11

13 Genetic Control of Immunity

GENES CONTROLLING THE IMMUNE RESPONSE — 13.1
MHC LINKED IMMUNE RESPONSE GENES — 13.1
LEVEL OF ACTION OF IMMUNE RESPONSE GENES — 13.3
    Antigen Presentation and T/B Cooperation 13.3, Cytotoxic T Cells 13.4
ANTIGEN RECOGNITION BY T CELLS AND B CELLS — 13.6
    Immune Response to HEL 13.6, Cross-Reactive Idiotypes 13.7
NON-MHC IMMUNE RESPONSE GENES — 13.8
GENETICALLY IMMUNODEFICIENT MOUSE STRAINS — 13.8
    B Cell Defects 13.8, Models of Autoimmune Disease 13.9
DEVELOPMENT OF THE GENES OF THE IMMUNE SYSTEM — 13.9

14 Development of the Immune System

LYMPHOID CELLS — 14.1
    T Cells 14.2, B Cells 14.4
DEVELOPMENT OF CLASS DIVERSITY — 14.5
DEVELOPMENT OF ANTIBODY DIVERSITY — 14.6
DEVELOPMENT OF MONONUCLEAR PHAGOCYTES AND ANTIGEN-PRESENTING CELLS — 14.7
THE COMPLEMENT SYSTEM — 14.7
DEVELOPMENT OF NEUTROPHIL FUNCTIONS — 14.7

15 Evolution of Immunity

INVERTEBRATE IMMUNITY — 15.1
    Immunocytes 15.1, 'Lymphoid' Tissues 15.2, Cell-Mediated Immunity 15.2, Non-Specific Defence 15.3
VERTEBRATE IMMUNITY — 15.4
    T and B Functions 15.4
MORPHOLOGY OF LYMPHOID TISSUES IN LOWER VERTEBRATES — 15.5
    Thymus 15.5, Spleen 15.6, Lymphomyeloid Nodes 15.6, Gut-Associated Lymphoid Tissue 15.7, Kidney 15.7, Bone Marrow 15.7
ASPECTS OF AMPHIBIAN IMMUNOLOGY — 15.8
    Thymus Development: *Xenopus laevis* 15.8, Alloimmunity: *Rana pipiens* 15.9, Immunoglobulin Production 15.10, Metamorphosis and Immunoregulation 15.10, Models for the Study of Lymphocyte Development 15.10

16 Immunity to Viruses, Bacteria and Fungi

IMMUNITY TO VIRUSES — 16.1
    Viral Infection 16.2, Effects of Antibody 16.3, Antibody Dependent Cell-Mediated Cytotoxicity 16.4, Cytotoxic T Cells and MHC Restriction 16.4, Delayed Hypersensitivity to Viral Antigens 16.5, Interferon 16.5, Immunopathology 16.6
IMMUNITY TO BACTERIA — 16.6
    Bacterial Cell Walls 16.6, Adjuvanticity and Other Non-Specific Mechanisms 16.7, The Role of Antibody 16.8, Interaction with Phagocytes 16.9, The Killing Mechanisms of Polymorphs and Macrophages – Non-Oxygen-Dependent 16.9, Oxygen-Dependent Killing Mechanisms 16.10, Defence Mechanisms in Bacterial Infection 16.10
IMMUNITY TO FUNGI — 16.11